F*CK
YOURSELF
FIT

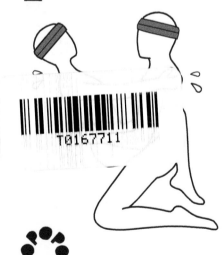

POP PRESS

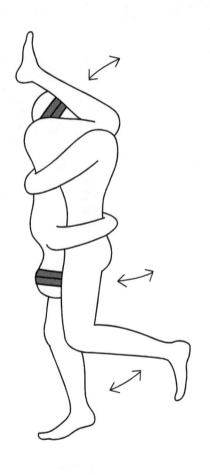

CONTENTS

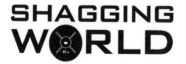

SHAGGING
WORLD

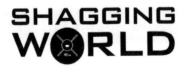

SHAGGING WORLD

CUM ON IN — TO SHAGGING WORLD

We're the nation's most popular intercourse-based fitness programme, helping thousands of people every week turn fat into fine through fucking. Our state-of-the-art gyms and intimate groups can be found all over the country – just look out for the Shagging World logo outside our venues.

Community is a big part of what we do. After all, we're not called Wanking World. If you don't arrive with a partner, you can download the Shagging World app so you can swipe away until you find your perfect workout mate. And, if all else fails, we have the patented Shagging World sexercise doll, available in a variety of shapes, sizes, colours and genders to ensure you get maximum results.

You'll find everything you need at our gym bars: post-workout shakes, condoms and lube, and the latest Shagging World clobber, such as our

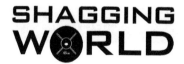

SHAGGING WORLD

transparent lacy sports bras and crotchless running shorts. We also have onsite personal trainers, sex therapists and video analysts to dissect your performance. Because at Shagging World, you know we've got you covered.

This book will give you the tools you need to maintain your progress outside of our gyms and group sessions. By following these home/public space sexercises, you'll earn Sins for exertion levels – to spend on indulgences such as a box set binge or a much-needed effort-free wank – and Sex Points – which reward your sexual adventurism – to keep you motivated so that you'll soon have the body you always dreamed of.

So go on, fly the Shagging World logo at full mast outside your home and get going with the nation's most popular intercourse-based fitness plan: *it's time to fuck yourself fit.*

SEX POINTS

50

CUMFORT ZONE
You've earned yourself a T-shirt bearing the logo
I came @ Shagging World

100

FAT-BURNING ZONE
Our patented Shagging World crotchless running shorts are yours.

200

CARDIO ZONE
Have a seven-day Shagging Plan and some 1-2-1 attention from our very personal trainers on us.

500

HOT AND HEAVY ZONE
Congratulations! You've got our portable Shag-replacement Kit: for those days when you don't have a partner but you still want to feel the burn.

1000

FUCKED YOURSELF WELL FIT ZONE
Have a year's free membership on us. And maybe an ice bath for your genitals.

SINS

50
- Box set binge
- Glass of booze
- Bar of chocolate

100
- Cheat day (not on your partner)
- Non-sexercise wank/shag
- Bottle of booze

150
- A good cry
- Box set weekend (getting dressed = optional)
- Three chocolate bars, to be eaten at once

200
- Eat-your-feelings evening
- Cocktails!
- All the crisps

250
- Recovery/celibate week
- Your own bodyweight in booze
- Enough chocolate to furnish several Easters

The Saddle Straddle

Studies have shown the benefits of sexercise on mental health – as well as on developing a great ass. **Yee-haw!**

 30 MINUTES

 200 CALORIES

 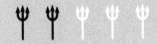

 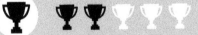

Abs, Ass

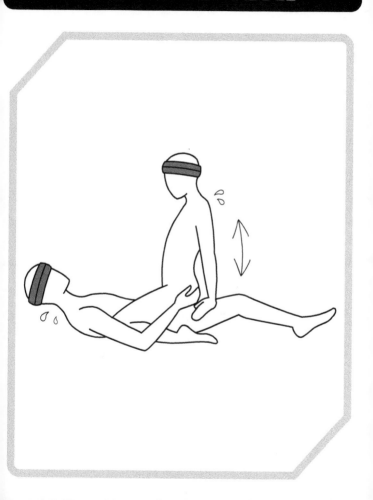

THE REVERSE SADDLE STRADDLE

PLAN ON STAYING **IN THE SADDLE** FOR AS LONG AS YOU CAN WITH THIS STONE-COLD CLASSIC FROM THE SHAGGING WORLD SEXERCISE BANK.

 20 MINUTES

 150 CALORIES

 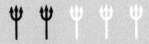

 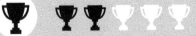

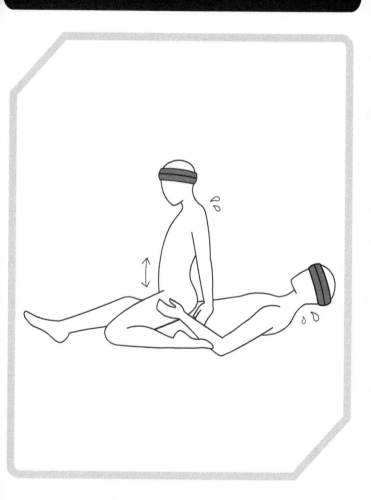

SLAM DUNKER

A PERFECT POSE FOR BOTH A DEEP STRETCH AND DEEP ENTRY, THE SLAM DUNKER IS A SURE THING TO GUARANTEE THAT TAKING CARE OF YOUR BODY IS ALWAYS A DEEPLY PLEASURABLE EXPERIENCE.

 10 MINUTES

 60 CALORIES

 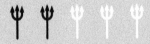

 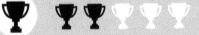

ABS, ASS

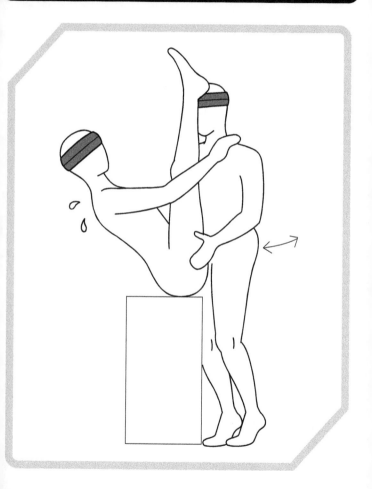

LEVITATOR

TAKE YOUR FITNESS PROGRAMME TO A HIGHER PLANE WITH THE LEVITATOR — AND IF YOU HAVE TO COME CRASHING BACK TO EARTH, DO SO IN THE KNOWLEDGE THAT YOU'VE FUCKED YOURSELF INTO FAR FINER SHAPE THAN WHEN YOU LEFT THE GROUND.

 5 MINUTES

 100 CALORIES

 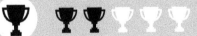

Abs, Ass

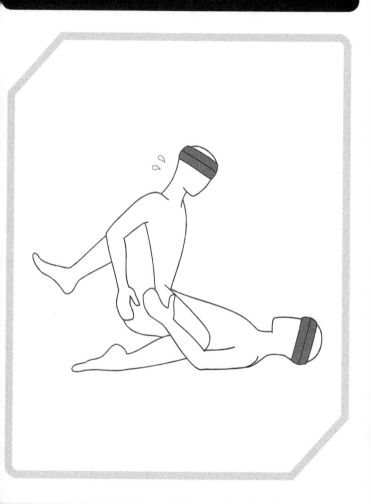

LAPS

This is how we run our laps at Shagging World. A long and slow pose for the endurance athletes among you. It might feel cramped in there but you'll want to make sure you don't get cramp as you head towards the home straight.

 25 Minutes (or as long as you can go)

 110 calories

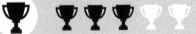

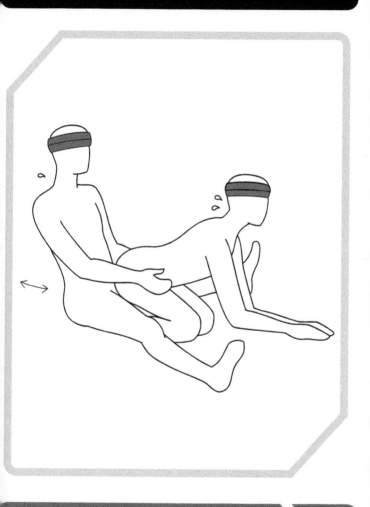

ABS-OLUTELY FABULOUS

BRING COITUS TO YOUR CRUNCHES AND 'JUST ONE MORE REP' MIGHT CUM SO MUCH EASIER THAN YOU IMAGINED.

 20 CRUNCHES, THEN REST AND REPEAT

 50 PER 20 CRUNCHES

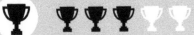

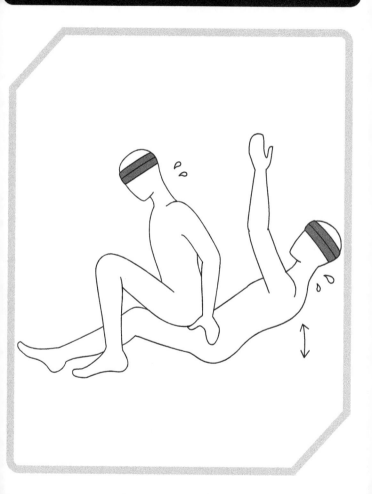

ROLY-POLY RUMPY-PUMPY

REDISCOVER YOUR INNER CHILD WITH YOUR ROLY-POLY AS YOU COME TO TERMS WITH YOUR OUTER ADULT IN A POSE THAT IS ANYTHING BUT INNOCENT.

 5 MINUTES

 75 CALORIES

 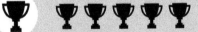 ABS, ASS

ROLY-POLY RUMPY-PUMPY

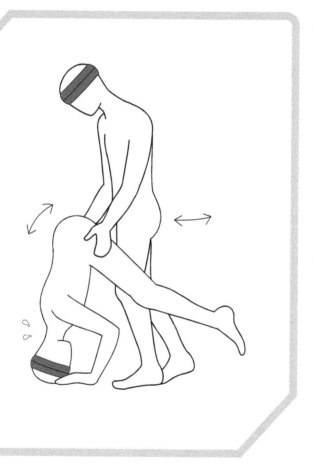

X LEG-OVER

No star-crossed lovers, please, just crossed legs and an insatiable thirst for bodily improvement through sexercise. It will take a lot more than fate to stop you getting the bod you crave.

 5 MINUTES

 75 CALORIES

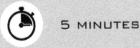

ABS, ASS

X LEG-OVER

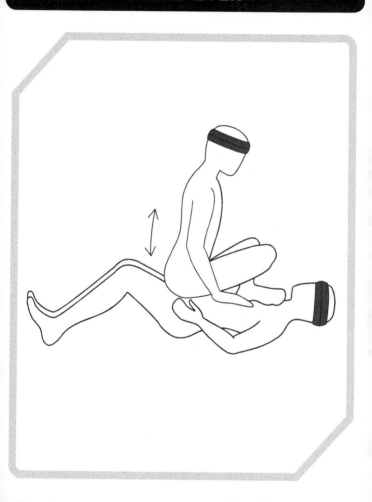

SQUAT GOBBLER

Squat then straighten those legs for the ultimate burn while delivering ultimate pleasure to your Shagging World partner. (Their turn next!)

 20 REPS

 40 CALORIES

 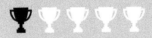

Abs, Ass

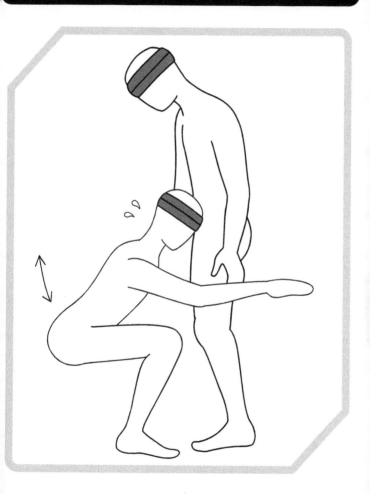

Abs, Ass

THE BACK-BEND BONK

LET YOUR PARTNER ADMIRE YOUR TRULY MAGNIFICENT ARCH FOR THE FULLY ALLOTTED TIME – JUST DON'T GO COLLAPSING WHEN THE CLIMAX IS IN SIGHT!

 5 MINUTES

 80 CALORIES

ABS, ASS

THE BACK-BEND BONK

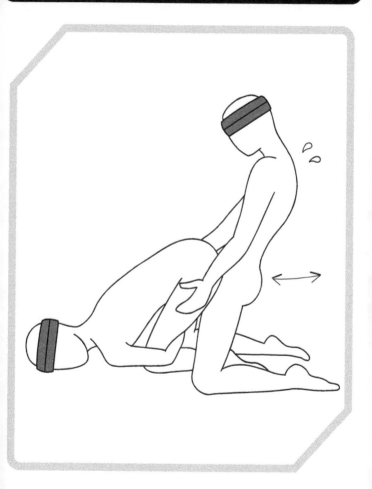

CORE BLIMEY!

THIS 2-LEGGED DOG KNOWS HOW TO GET UP AND PLEASE — AND WORK YOUR CORE 4 SURE.

 5 MINUTES

 100 CALORIES

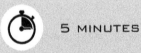

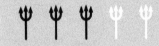

 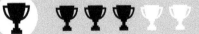

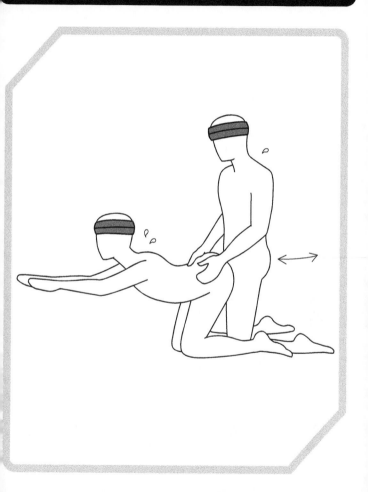

THE PASSION POUCH

Strength, poise and desire are just some of the qualities you'll need to deliver a textbook Passion Pouch. Remember, practice — and lots of it — makes perfect.

 5 MINUTES

 100 CALORIES

 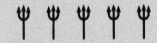

 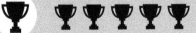

LEGS, ASS

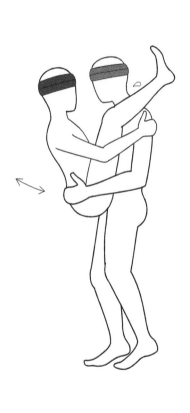

WALKING THE DOG

WALK THIS DOGGY AND REAP THE
EXTRA BURN OF A CLASSIC POSITION.
CARPET BURN OBLIGATORY. KNEE
PADS OPTIONAL FOR HARD FLOORS.

 10 MINUTES

 125 CALORIES

 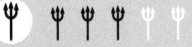

 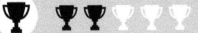

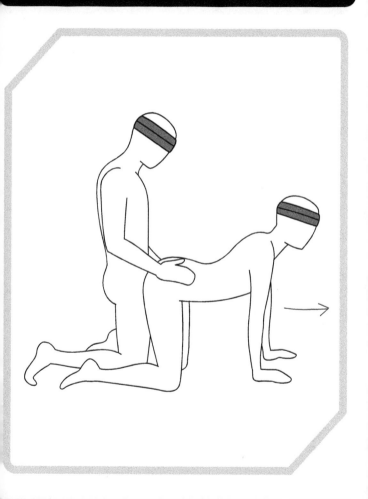

ANOTHER HAMSTRING TO YOUR BLOW

The Shagging World warm-up technique of choice to stretch those strings and stir your juices.

 ONE MINUTE PER HAMSTRING (REPEAT AS DESIRED)

 40 CALORIES

 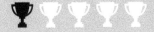

ANOTHER HAMSTRING TO YOUR BLOW

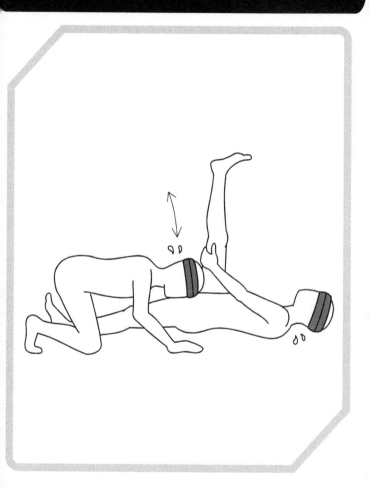

THE ELEVATOR

RIDE THIS **ELEVATOR** ALL THE WAY UP TO THE HEAVENTH FLOOR – AND THEN BACK AGAIN.

 5 MINUTES

 90 CALORIES

 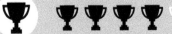

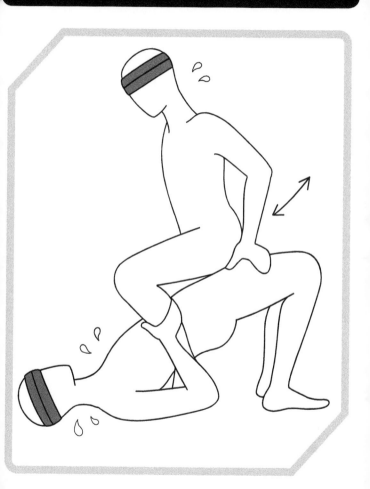

THE HELLS BELLS BEND

You'll quickly find that there's no wrong angle as you attempt to make a right angle to penetrate.

 10 MINUTES

 120 CALORIES

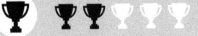

LEGS, ASS

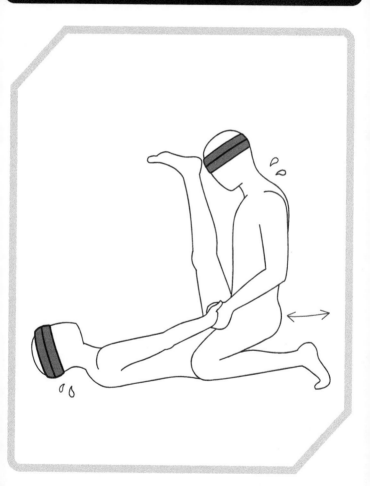

TUCKY FUCKY

THE TIGHTER THE TUCK, THE BETTER THE FUCK — AND THE HARDER THE WORKOUT. BEND DEEP AND SHAG HARD WITH THE TUCKY FUCKY.

 10 MINUTES

 95 CALORIES

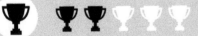 LEGS, ASS

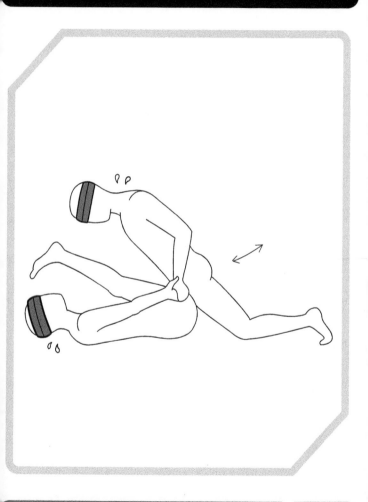

FLAMINGO LAND

Make like the feathery pink ones on one leg as you form your own attraction in the Shagging World theme park.

 5 MINS PER LEG

 95 CALORIES

 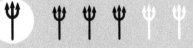

 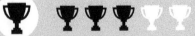

LEGS, ASS

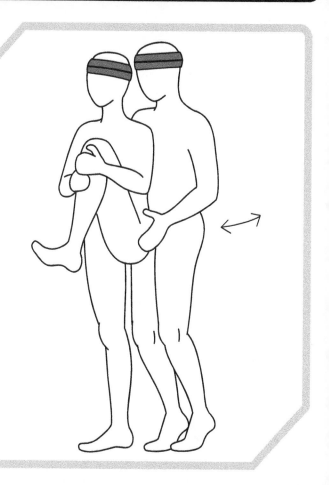

Do It by Calves

Why do it by halves when you can Do It by Calves for the ultimate burn?

2 MINS PER CALF
(REPEAT AS DESIRED)

40+ CALORIES

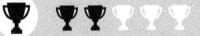

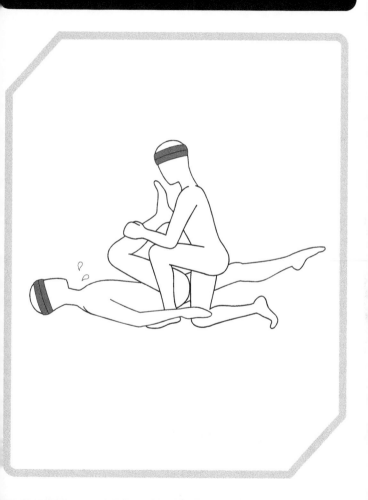

SEX SQUAT

Sometimes the best names for a pose are also the most literal. This is sex. This is a squat. This is Sex Squat. You're welcome.

 5 MINUTES

 65 CALORIES

 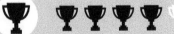

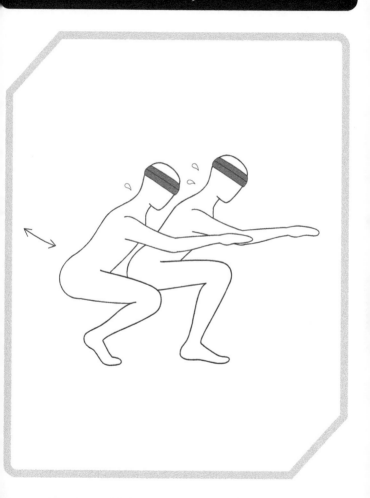

TOUCH THE SKY

IT MIGHT SOUND STRANGE TO TOUCH YOUR TOES WHEN YOU'RE REACHING FOR THE HEAVENS, BUT GIVE THIS ONE A GO — OH, OH, OH — AND IT WILL ALL CUM CLEAR.

 5 MINUTES

 45 CALORIES

 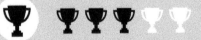

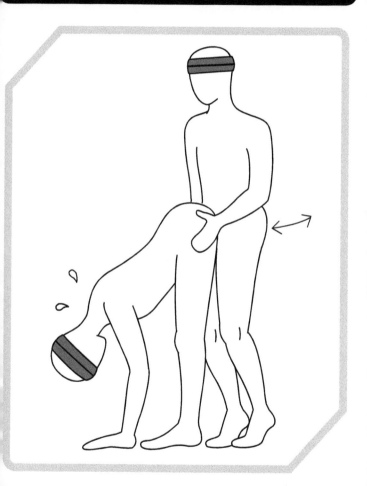

SPREAD EAGLE

HOLD THAT POSE EVEN AS YOUR PARTNER HAS YOU FEELING LIKE YOU'RE SOARING LIKE AN EAGLE IN THE STRATOSPHERE OF YOUR PERSONAL PLEASUREDOME. YOUR HAMSTRINGS WILL THANK YOU FOR IT.

 10 MINUTES

 40 CALORIES

 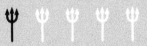

 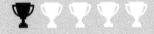

LEGS, ASS

SPREAD EAGLE

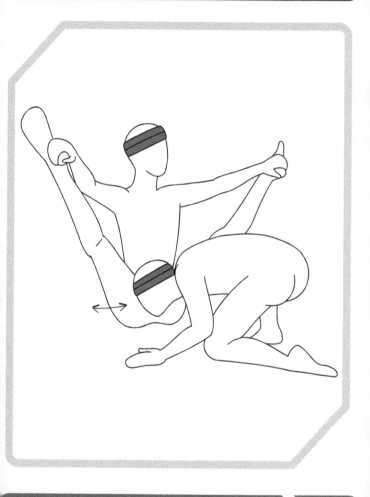

LUNGE PLUNGE

Take the plunge with this patented Shagging World variation on the classic lunge and feel the burn – then swap legs and take another turn.

 10 minutes – 5 on each leg

 60 calories

 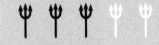

 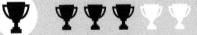

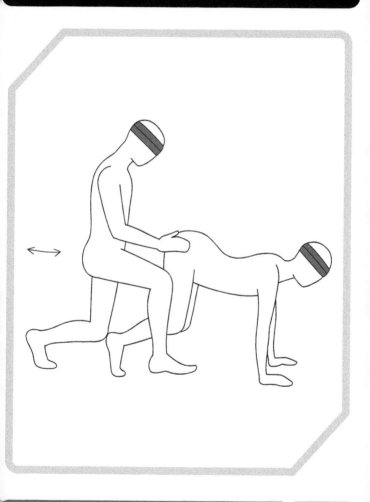

BUCKAROO BONKO

RIDE AS LONG AS YOU CAN BEFORE IT'S TIME TO **BUCKAROO!**

 5 MINUTES

 150 CALORIES

 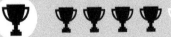

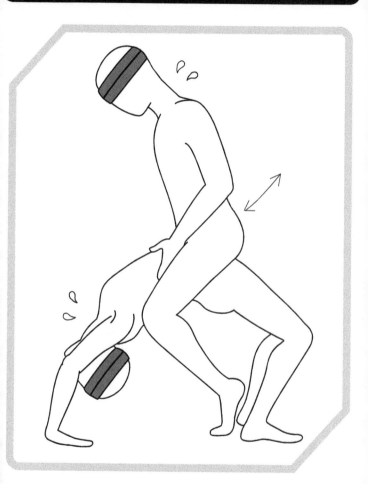

CART BEFORE THE HORSE

THE SISTER MOVE TO CORE BLIMEY, YOU'LL HAVE CARTE BLANCHE TO **RIDE THIS CART** HOWEVER YOU SEE FIT.

 20 MINUTES

 150 CALORIES

 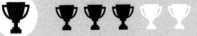

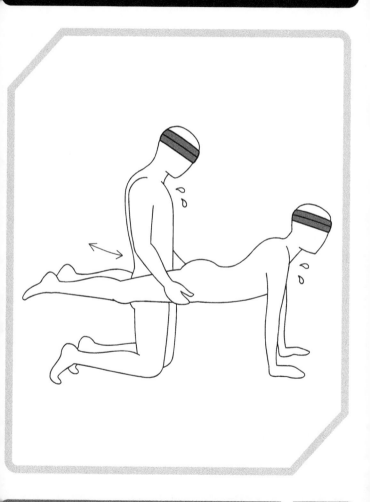

THE OVERHEAD HEAD PRESS

When the weight you're lifting over your head is actually a person, you're also simulating to climax? That's sexercise, the Shagging World way, my friend.

 10 REPS

 120 CALORIES

 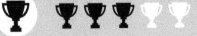

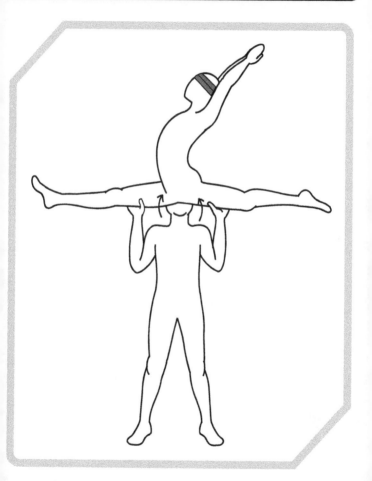

THE HENCH PRESS

Hench Press your partner as they give you head. Can you reach the climax of your reps before you, well, climax all over your partner's face?

 20 REPS

 95 CALORIES

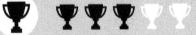

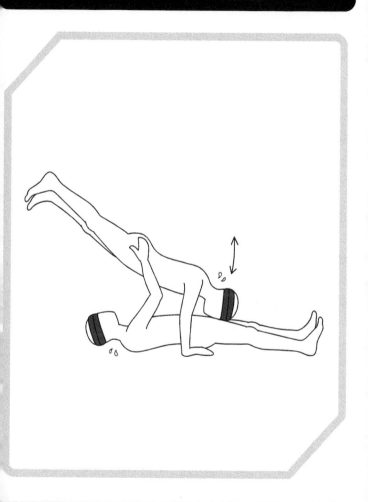

ANKLE GRABS

Lean back, grab your partner's ankles, spread your legs and enjoy this wildly liberating pose. The question on every Shagging World member's lips: Have you done your ankle grabs today?

 10 MINUTES

 100 CALORIES

 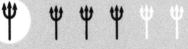

 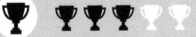

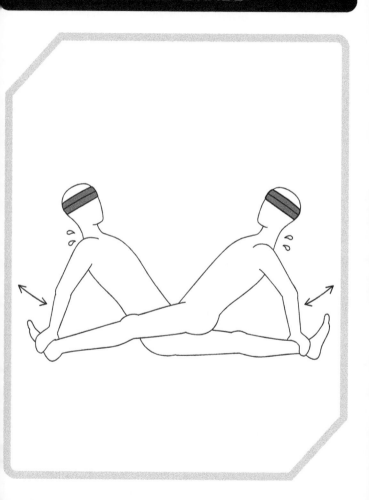

THE HIGH ROAD

You take the High Road, while your partner takes the low road (and sends you higher and higher).

 5 MINUTES

 60 CALORIES

 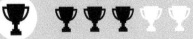

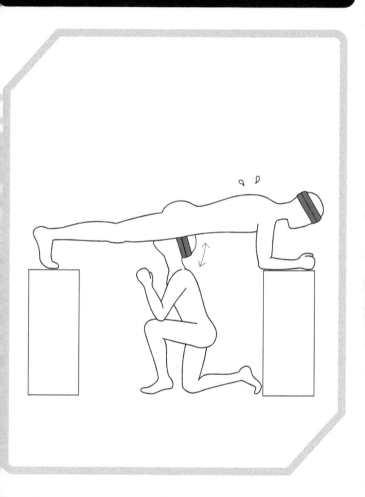

PUMP UPS

Not just a press up. Not just pumping hot love your partner's way. These are Pump Ups, a Shagging World classic to get the arms, pecs and pecker primed.

 20 PUMP UPS, THEN REST AND REPEAT

 60 PER 20 PUMP UPS

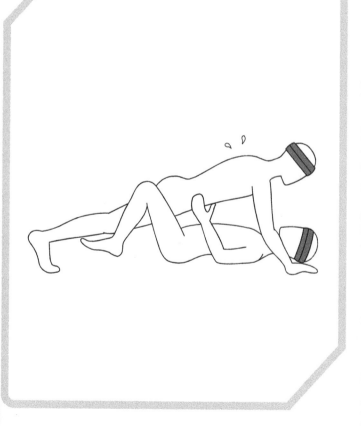

PUMP UPS (THE VOLUME)

LIKE THE PUMP UPS, BUT HARDER, HARDER, HARDER, AND LOUDER, LOUDER, LOUDER. BAD NEWS FOR YOUR NEIGHBOURS, THOUGH AT SHAGGING WORLD GYMS WE HAVE OUR POUNDING DANCE MUSIC RAMPED SO EAR-BLEEDINGLY HIGH, YOU WON'T HEAR A THING. POSSIBLY FOR HOURS AFTERWARDS.

 20 PUMP UPS (THE VOLUME)

 90 PER 20 PUMPS UPS (THE VOLUME)

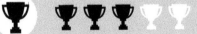

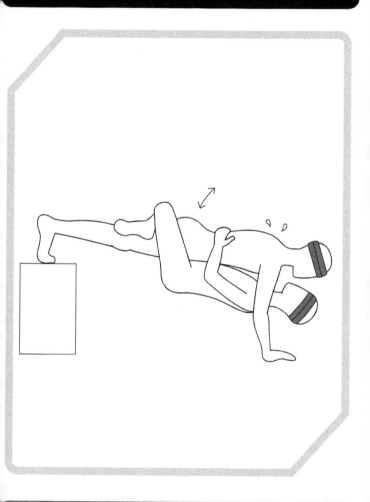

FLYING CARPET

THERE'S SOMETHING TRULY MAGICAL ABOUT THIS POSE, WHICH WILL WORK YOUR BODY LIKE YOU WOULDN'T BELIEVE — AND TAKE YOU SOARING TO PLACES YOU MIGHT THINK BELONG IN FAIRY TALES.

 5 MINUTES

 80 CALORIES

 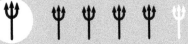

 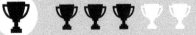

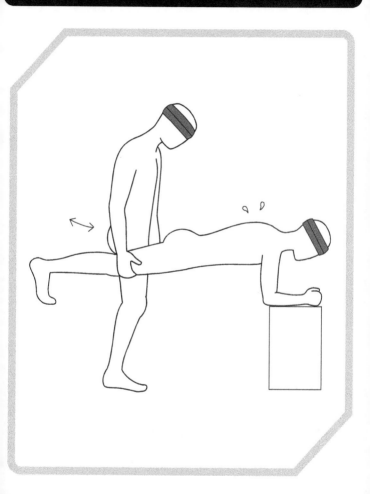

HEAVENLY HAND-STANDS

UPSIDE-DOWN ORGASMS ARE JUST THE TONIC FOR THE MIND, BODY AND SOUL. SHAGGING WORLD STRONGLY ADVISES USING A WALL FOR BALANCE, AND WILL NOT BE HELD RESPONSIBLE FOR THE CONSEQUENCES OF ANY MID-COITUS COLLAPSE.

 4 MINUTES

 95 CALORIES

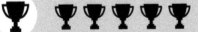

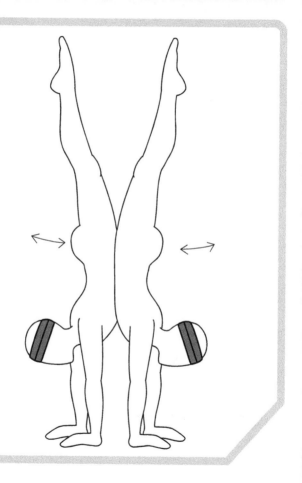

HORNY HAND PLANT

Your arms and ass are going to love you for this one, and your Shagging World partner won't be entirely unhappy with you either.

 5 MINUTES

 85 CALORIES

 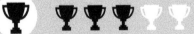

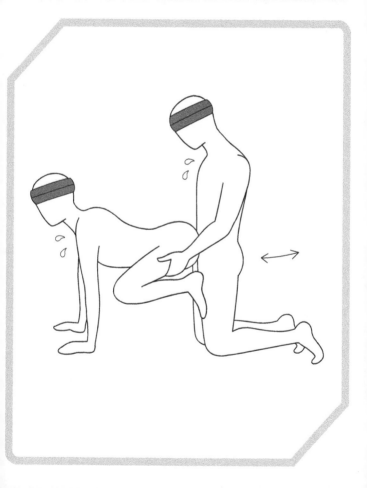

'HEAD' STAND

Here at Shagging World, we always say that a bog-standard handstand is a waste of a perfectly good set of genitals. Do the anything-but-yogic Head Stand and find out why we have no end of satisfied members.

 2 MINUTES

 45 CALORIES

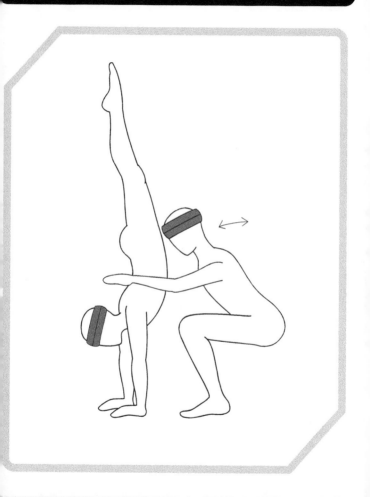

SPACE WALK

SLIP ON THE ANTI-GRAVITY BOOTS AND PREPARE TO GIVE HEAD AS YOUR OWN HEAD SEES LIFE ON EARTH — OR AT LEAST YOUR PARTNER'S GENITALS — FROM A DIFFERENT PERSPECTIVE.

 5 MINUTES

 95 CALORIES

 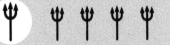

 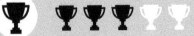

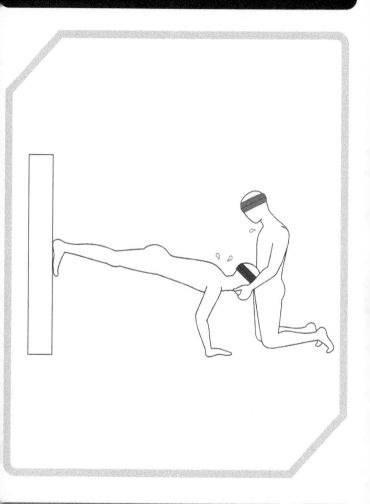

EASY RIDER

You'll find this pose anything but easy as you try to maintain form while your partner rides you into the ground. Don't fall short at the final hurdle...

 10 MINUTES

 90 CALORIES

 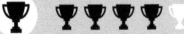

CHEST, BACK, SOME ASS

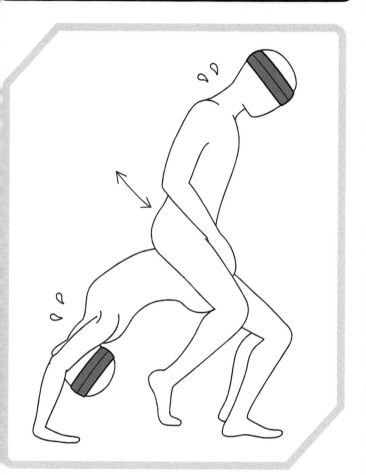

Mighty Members

A Shagging World fave named in honour of our mighty members — and, of course, any other kinds of 'member' involved. In case that isn't clear, we mean dicks.

 5 minutes

 90 calories

 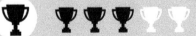

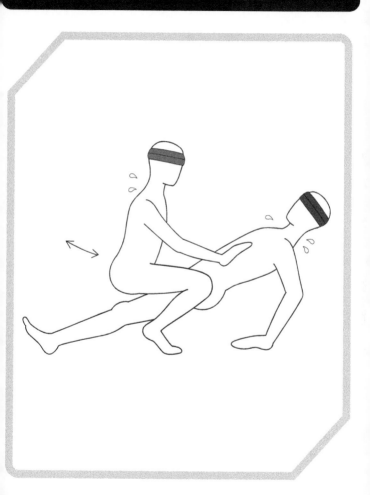

SIT UP AND BEG

THE ONLY KIND OF SEXUAL BEGGING PERMITTED IN SHAGGING WORLD GYMS (COME ON, PEOPLE, DIGNITY PLEASE!), THIS POSE WILL LEAVE YOU BEGGING FOR MORE, THOUGH, AS JUST STATED, THAT'S NOT ACTUALLY PERMITTED IN OUR GYMS. INTERNALISE IT.

 10 MINUTES

 100 CALORIES

 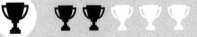

　CHEST, BACK, SOME ASS

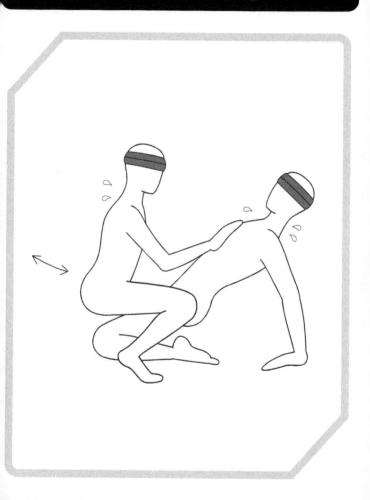

THE WALL MOUNT

A FIVE-MINUTE STAND-UP SHAG BURNS MORE CALORIES THAN YOU'D REAP AT A STAND-UP DESK ALL DAY, SO WHY WASTE YOUR TIME? SIT DOWN AT WORK AND STAND UP FOR YOUR SHAG.

 5 MINUTES

 75 CALORIES

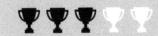

* 3 IN A PRIVATE PLACE, 4 IN A PUBLIC SPACE, OR 5 IF YOU MANAGE THE WALL MOUNT AT WORK.

THE WALL MOUNT

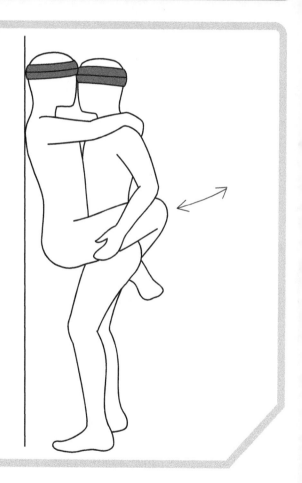

PILE DRIVER

A favourite of Shagging World veterans and A&E doctors alike – **SHAG SAFE** with this one, loyal subscribers.*

*(Shagging World will not be held responsible in the event of any accident or injury.)

 5 MINUTES

 150 CALORIES

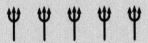

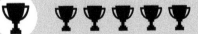

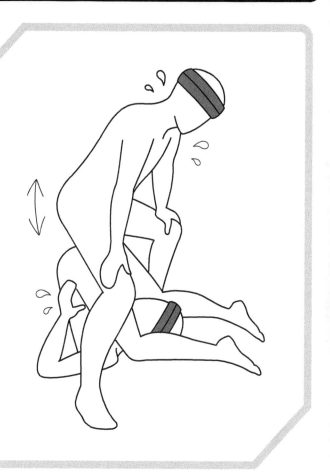

69 FOR TWO MINUTES, THEN SWITCH TO PENETRATION OF YOUR CHOICE, THEN BACK TO 69, AND SO ON ... Shagging World is proud to produce its own brand of mouthwash for between 'courses', should you desire.

 4 + MINUTES

 120 + CALORIES

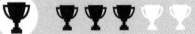 CHEST, BACK, SOME ASS

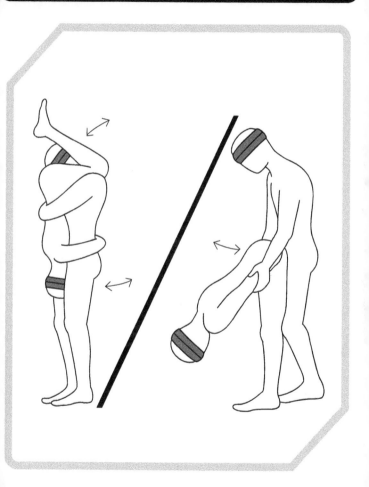

BACK-BEND BANQUET

CHOW DOWN ON WHAT IS ESSENTIALLY A CALORIE-FREE FEAST WHILE YOUR PARTNER RACKS UP THE SINS AND SEX POINTS.

 10 MINUTES

 85 CALORIES

 🔱🔱🔱🔱🔱

 🏆🏆🏆🏆🏆

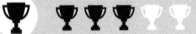

BACK-BEND BANQUET

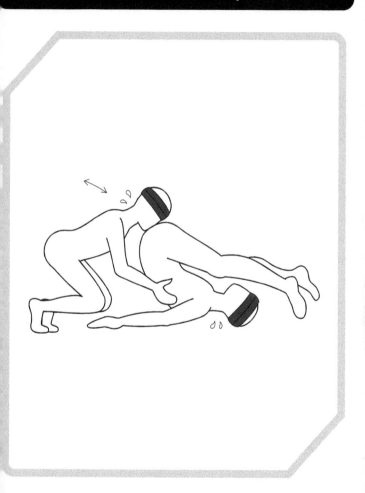

HITTING THE WALL

ATHLETES TALK ABOUT HITTING THE WALL — BUT THEY RARELY HAVE THE LUXURY OF A RIM JOB AND A HAND JOB APPLIED SIMULTANEOUSLY TO KEEP THEM GOING. MAKE SURE YOU HIT THE SWEET SPOT BEFORE YOU BUCKLE UNDER YOUR PARTNER.

 5 MINUTES

 95 CALORIES

 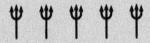

 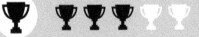

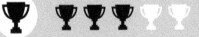

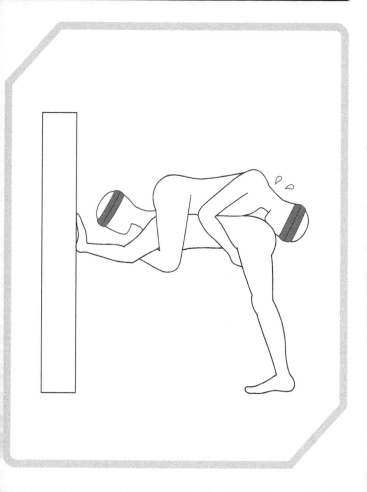

DIRTY BURPEE

THE ONLY BURPEE YOU'RE EVER LIKELY TO WILLINGLY REPEAT IN YOUR LIFE, YOU'LL FUCK YOURSELF FIT IN NO TIME WITH THIS POSE.

10 MINS +
(1 MIN IN EACH POSITION, REPEATED 5 TIMES OR MORE)

150 + CALORIES

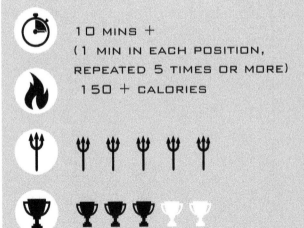

DIRTY BURPEE

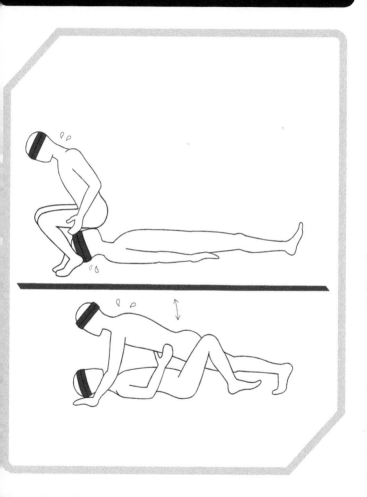

FLATLINER

You'll need to be flexible to be a **Flatliner**, but know your limitations: a bend in the legs is better than a berth on a stretcher, after all.

 50 MINUTES

 70 CALORIES

 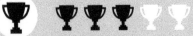

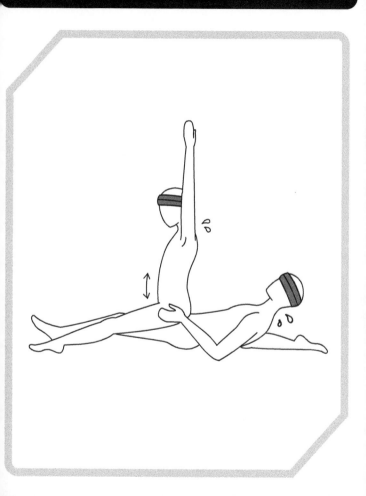

TWIST AND SHOUT

CUM ON, CUM ON, CUM ON BABY NOW, LET'S WORK OUT! STRENGTH, POISE AND GRACE (POSSIBLY) COMBINED WITH AN INSATIABLE SEXUAL THIRST TO GET FIT COULD SEE YOUR TWIST AND SHOUT BECOME A SCREAM OF PURE PLEASURE.

 5 MINUTES

 95 CALORIES

 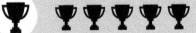

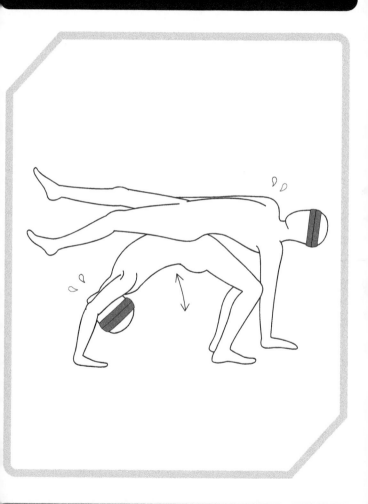

SEXY STIRRUPS

Your feet won't touch the ground as you ride for your life — well, your hot bod, at any rate — in the Sexy Stirrups.

 5 MINUTES

 140 CALORIES

 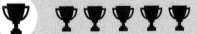

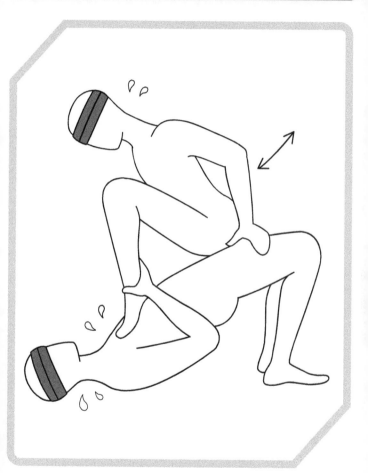

SEATED 69

THE PUNCHLINE FOR THIS POSE IS THAT THERE IS NO SEAT: SQUAT AND HOLD — AND TRY TO MAKE SURE YOU BOTH CUM BEFORE YOU COLLAPSE!

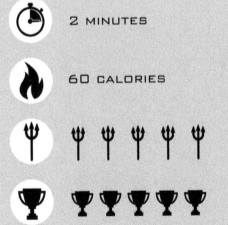

2 MINUTES

60 CALORIES

THE WHOLE SHEBANG

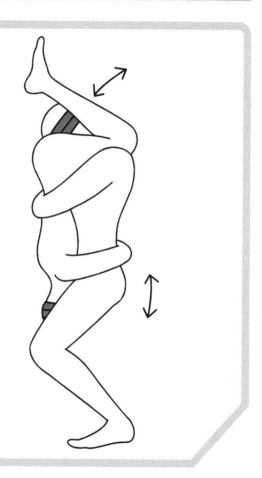

HEAD TO TOE

A TANGLE OF LIMBS THAT WOULD MAKE A RENDITION OF 'HEAD, SHOULDERS, KNEES AND TOES' HARD WORK, BUT THANKFULLY WILL ALLOW YOU TO DO ALL THE WORK TO GET HARD AND GET HENCH.

 10 MINUTES

 150 CALORIES

 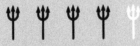

 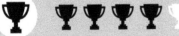

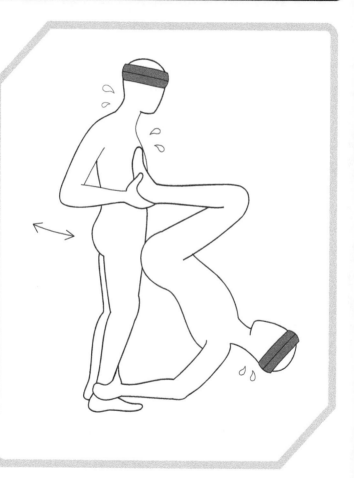

TANTRIC TRIANGLES

MAKE LIKE A THREE-SIDED SHAPE AS YOU ATTEMPT TWO-SIDED PLEASURE. RIGHT ANGLES ARE OPTIONAL, BUT MAKE SURE YOU HAVE THE RIGHT ANGLE FOR ENTRY.

 5 MINUTES

 130 CALORIES

 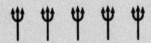

 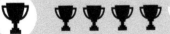

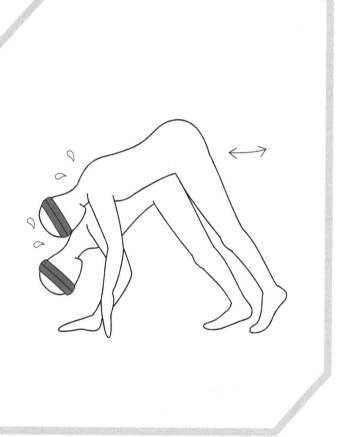

THE ROWING MACHINE

Depending on the gender makeup of your couple, you could be a surefire cert for glory in the coxless pairs or simply delighted to stick your oar in. Either way, row safely!

 10 MINUTES

 160 CALORIES

 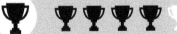

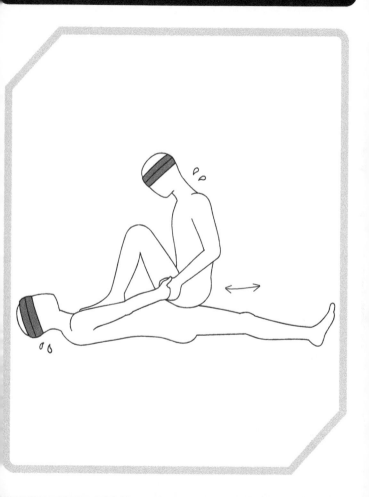

SIDE SWIPE

A BALANCING ACT SURE TO BEAR
FRUIT IN THE FORM OF ARM MUSCLES
AND UPPER BODY STRENGTH — AND
HOPEFULLY A BLISTERING FINISH
BEFORE COLLAPSING IN A HEAP.

 5 MINUTES

 120 CALORIES

 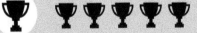

SIDE SWIPE

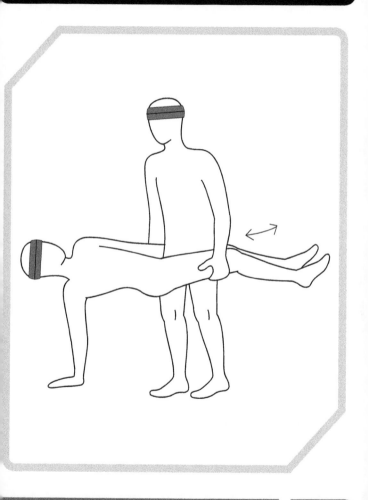

CLIMBING THE WALLS

LIKE ANY GOOD CLIMBER, YOU KNOW THE RISKS INHERENT IN WHAT YOU'RE DOING. SO, YOU KNOW, DON'T FALL AND REMEMBER TO WEAR PROTECTION.

 5 MINUTES

 90 CALORIES

 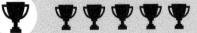

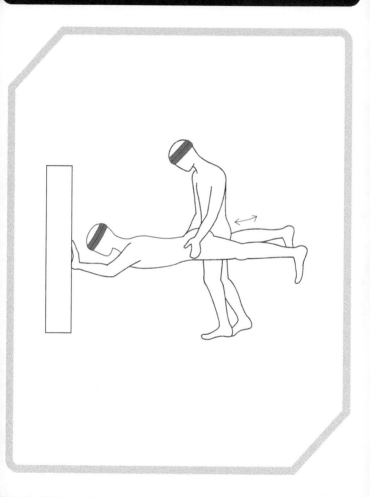

THE RACY RACE

ON YOUR MARKS, GET SET, GO!
RUNNING ON THE SPOT TO THE KIND
OF POUNDING MUSIC ON ENDLESS
REPEAT IN SHAGGING WORLD GYMS
MAKES THIS THE RACIEST RACE
YOU'RE EVER LIKELY TO TAKE PART
IN BEFORE BREAKFAST.

 2 MINUTES

 120 CALORIES

 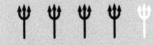

 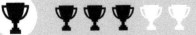

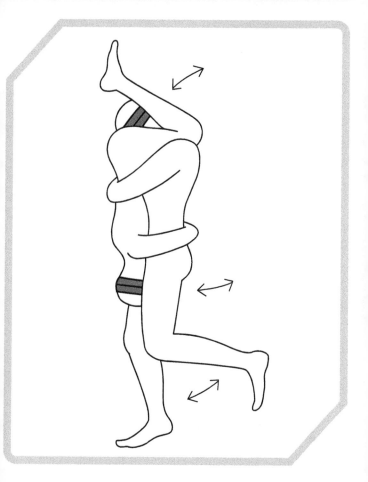

BOTTOM'S UP

Not just good for your ass — the Bottom's Up will take good care of your arms and core too. Something we can all drink to, I'm sure. (Protein shake or smoothie recommended.)

 10 MINUTES

 110 CALORIES

 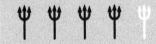

 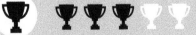

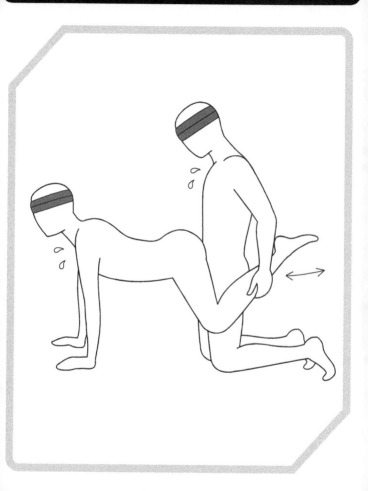

X-TASY

Cartwheel your way into a better tomorrow, and try not to let all the blood rush to your head as you're given head.

 5 MINUTES

 95 CALORIES

 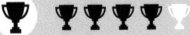

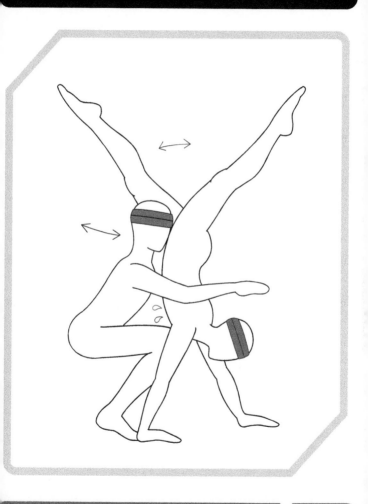

HEAD OVER HEELS

Forget the 'L' word — it's a far better workout for your heart to do this version of Head Over Heels. (Falling in love optional and not directly encouraged among Shagging World members.)

 5 MINUTES

 150 CALORIES

 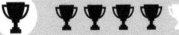

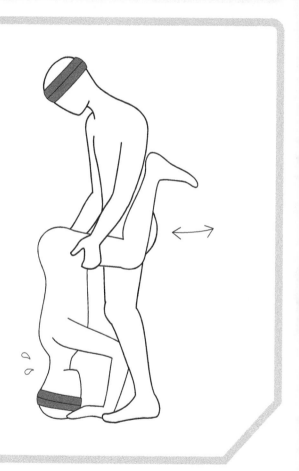

MARATHON MAN
(WOMAN, OR ANY GENDER IDENTITY)

THE WORLD RECORD FOR THE MARATHON IS 2 HOURS, 1 MINUTE AND 18 SECONDS. YOU'LL WANT TO CONSERVE ENERGY, TAP INTO THAT TANTRA AND TAKE TURNS ON TOP IF YOU'RE GOING TO GO FOR THAT LONG.

 2 HOURS, 1 MINUTE AND 18 SECONDS +

 750 +

 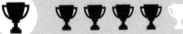

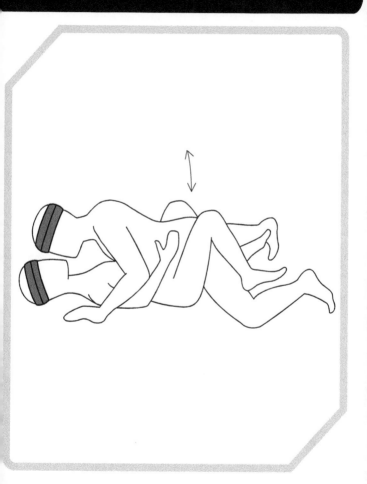

HORNY HIPS

Control is the key word here, if you want to maximise the benefits to your leg muscles – and, of course, not serve yourself short in the pleasure department.

 10 MINS (5 ON EACH SIDE)

 90 CALORIES

 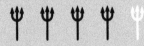

 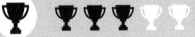

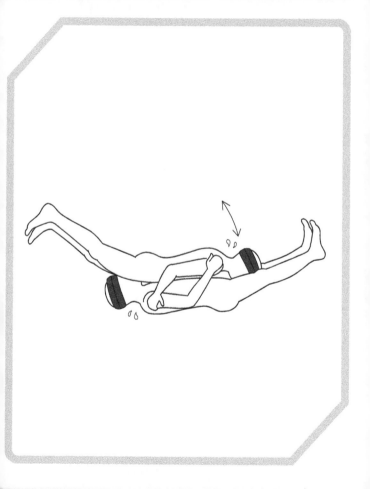

Pop Press, an imprint of Ebury Publishing,
20 Vauxhall Bridge Road,
London SW1V 2SA

Pop Press is part of the Penguin Random House group of companies
whose addresses can be found at global.penguinrandomhouse.com

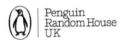

Penguin
Random House
UK

First published in the United Kingdom by Pop Press in 2020

www.penguin.co.uk

A CIP catalogue record for this book is available from the
British Library

ISBN 9781529107173
Design by Emily Snape
Shagging World copywriter: Steve Burdett
Project management by whitefox
Printed and bound in Great Britain by Clays Ltd, Elcograf S.p.A.

Penguin Random House is committed to a sustainable future for our
business, our readers and our planet. This book is made from Forest
Stewardship Council certified paper.

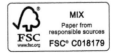

MIX
Paper from
responsible sources
FSC® C018179